Bye, Bye Cancer!

Bye, Bye Cancer!

A Simple, Effective Way to Prevent and Heal Cancer

Dr. Rhonda N. Cambridge-Phillip MD, MPH, HC

ISBN: 152375883X
ISBN 13: 9781523758838
Library of Congress Control Number: 2016903968
CreateSpace Independent Publishing Platform
North Charleston, South Carolina

This book is dedicated to the Most High, the Creator of all things. Without You, nothing is possible.

Dear God, You are my driving force. You keep me focused on gratitude, sharing, caring, and being of service to others. You push me to break out of the box and encourage me to step into my own spotlight and shine so, so brightly! Thank You for the great days and the good days. Thank You for the not-so-good days, which, looking back, made me so uncomfortable that I was forced to move upward and onward. I thank You and praise You for what You have done and for what You are about to do.

Amen.

CONTENTS

Acknowledgments

To MY MOM: thanks for always being my number-one fan.

To my older brother: I know you are watching me from heaven. I hope I make you proud.

To my other brother: thanks for teaching me the power of prayer.

To my husband: thanks for teaching me what it means to have a free spirit, something I am learning to master.

To my kids: I am so proud that I get to be your mom. You inspire me every single day to lead by example and be great.

Thanks to my other family members and many friends, who are like family because you show up and are present whenever I need you. (You know who you are and what you mean to me.)

Thanks to my many patients and clients for entrusting me with your health and wellness over the years.

Thanks to you! Yes, you, the person who is reading this book right now. We may not know each other, but thanks for being you—an individual with an open mind and heart. Thanks for putting your health first and taking the steps necessary to achieve optimal health and wellness. I salute you!

PART 1

The Problem

Finding My Voice: The Evolution of This Book

*There is no greater agony than bearing
an untold story inside of you.*

—Maya Angelou

Here is my story, which has been untold until now.

Ever since I was about ten years old, it has been my dream to become a physician and work in the community where I was born and raised. When I graduated from medical school sixteen years ago, I was so excited about the opportunity to truly make a difference and have a positive impact on the health of others. However, several years into my career, I became very disgruntled with the direction my career was taking. Because I worked and lived in the same community I grew up in, I often saw my patients and their families outside of the hospital setting, at the local markets, shopping areas, church, and other places. Many of these people were those I had admired as I was growing up for their strength, courage, drive, and zest for life. It was hard for me to just stand by and watch as they got sick. It seemed as though I should be doing more to help. I was watching the slow decline of the health of my people.

The health of my community members is, based on available health statistics, considered very poor. One of the more common health issues I have been witnessing over the years is cancer of all different types. I wanted and needed to make a difference, so my first objective was to learn more. To do this, I decided to go back to school to obtain a master's degree in public health. During this time, I took a course in nutrition epidemiology and became very interested in nutrition and food in my community. The course helped me learn about the quality of food and how food and overall nutrition are related to health. To gain even more insight and credibility, I then decided to become a certified health coach.

One of my goals is to help people in my community prevent, heal, and keep cancer in remission using an excellent nutrition supplementation program. We are mostly people of Afro Caribbean descent—blacks who are from the Caribbean ourselves or who have parents or grandparents from the Caribbean and now live in the United States. In my community, there is very limited access to quality food. There's a vast difference between the types and quality of foods available here and those offered in neighboring communities not populated by persons of Afro-Caribbean descent and other people of color. In neighborhoods like mine, there is a plethora of fast-food restaurants—too many to count on one hand. When we are able to locate good food, it is often much more expensive. Here is an example. I may be able to get a full meal for my family at the local fast-food chain for twenty dollars. However, if I go to the local supermarket, that same twenty dollars will usually get me a lot less food, especially if I try to choose whole foods. It is cheaper to eat foods with low nutritional value. Even the fast-food restaurants are different in neighborhoods like mine. I find it strange that in my neighborhood, some fast-food chains do not offer healthier eating options, such as salads. However, when

I travel outside my neighborhood to areas that are not heavily populated by people of color, salads are offered.

One simple solution, you might think, would be to shop in the neighborhoods that have better-quality food. However, most of us cannot afford to spend the time and money to leave our community on a regular basis in search of quality, unprocessed foods that are free of chemicals, toxins, herbicides, and pesticides—foods that are truly organic and not genetically modified or engineered.

Although I was born and raised in Brooklyn, New York, my parents emigrated from the Caribbean islands of Trinidad and Tobago. So I understand all too well the Caribbean culture and belief systems. I also understand the cultural role that food plays in this community. People of Caribbean descent, like those of many other cultures, socialize around food. It is tough to ask us to commit long term to changing the way we cook and eat because we pride ourselves on being able to hold onto this part of our culture. The ability to preserve as many customs as possible makes the whole process of leaving your home to build a life elsewhere much easier.

It is also difficult for us to change from eating Caribbean staples and favorites. Here are some examples of such favorites:

- **Pelau**: a stew made with chicken or beef. The meat is seared in carmelized sugar or molasses and then simmered with rice, coconut milk, and pigeon peas. The dish is served with a salad that usually includes avocados.
- **Oil down**: a stew made with breadfruit, green bananas or plantains, dumplings, pig tail, various spices, coconut milk, and oil
- **Cow-heel soup**: a soup usually made from split peas that also contains dumplings, carrots, corn on the cob, potatoes, and other provisions, including plantains, bananas, yams, dasheen, and cow heel
- **Fried bake and saltfish**: bake is a fried dough that is eaten in place of bread. The saltfish is usually a salted codfish that is sautéed with onions, tomatoes, black pepper, and other spices.

We ate a certain way in the Caribbean and got great health outcomes. However, it often seems that when we come to the United States and eat the same way that we ate in our home country, we get adverse health outcomes. Many medical professionals tell us that our traditional way of eating is causing us to become sick.

Perhaps the explanation is not so simple. In the Caribbean, we are used to eating nutrient-rich foods that are high in protein, fat, fiber, and carbohydrates. We also eat lots of truly organic fruits and vegetables. In our new homes in the United States, these same foods may not be as healthy. Even when people in my community can afford the time and money to access better-quality foods, more and more research is showing that conventionally grown produce may contain pesticide residues, even when it is washed and peeled. In some instances, foods that are labeled "organic" still contain herbicides and pesticides due to contamination.

It's also hard for us to know if our food is genetically engineered or modified. Congress passed legislation, including the Safe and Accurate Food

Labeling Act of 2015 (nicknamed the DARK Act, for "Deny Americans the Right to Know"), that makes it legal to sell such foods without labeling them and bans individual states from requiring GMO labeling.

When it comes to the health issue of cancer, various lifestyle modifications are known to play a role in prevention and healing. These include avoiding known carcinogens, managing stress, employing effective coping skills, engaging in healthy physical activity, tending to one's emotional and spiritual health, and eating healthy foods. Even in the face of particularly toxic environments, limited access to nutrient-rich foods, and other challenges that I outline later in this book, I have witnessed firsthand how healthy lifestyle modifications and nutritional supplementation can be used to aid in the prevention and healing of cancer.

For my community and those similar, one solution is to supplement the diet with quality, comprehensive, well-balanced minerals and vitamins. Nutrition supplementation is an excellent way to bridge the gap between what we are supposed to be getting in our food and what we are actually getting. However, there are many kinds of nutritional supplements on the market, and not all of them are created equal. Because the market is saturated, many consumers are confused about which supplements to use, in what quantity, and how often. People are concerned, and rightfully so, about side effects of supplements and the possibility of harmful interactions with prescription medications. This book addresses all of these issues in the context of the unique Caribbean culture.

As a physician who understands it well, I have noticed a lack of consideration for the role that our Caribbean culture plays in our health challenges, particularly cancer. For communities of Afro-Caribbean descent, nutrition supplementation is not merely an option but a necessity. I believe it should be added to existing cancer-prevention and cancer-treatment programs. Although this book is written from an Afro-Caribbean perspective, America is a melting pot. Persons emigrating from other parts of the world, from other backgrounds and demographics, may find the information just as useful. Upon completion of this book, you will understand the important role that nutrition supplementation may play in healing and preventing cancer. You will also learn how to go about choosing quality supplements.

On a personal note, I have been considering writing this book for many years. However, fear got the best of me until now. I was afraid that this message would not be accepted, particularly by my own colleagues and the wider medical community. I was afraid that others would question my intent and attack my character. I was scared of being called a quack because this message does not always align with traditional medical-belief systems. However, I realize that I owe it to my community and the world to get this message out and let you, the reader, decide whether to accept it or not. So no more delays—let's get to it!

CHAPTER 1

CANCER 101: A SIMPLIFIED WAY OF UNDERSTANDING CANCER

CANCER IS THE term used to describe the process of abnormal, uncontrolled cell growth. The body is comprised of a group of organ systems, which are comprised of groups of tissues, which are comprised of cells. There are trillions of cells in our bodies.[1] Healthy cells have a specified amount of time to grow, develop, replicate, and die. In scientific terms, this is known as the "cell cycle." Normal, programmed cell death is called "apoptosis." Cancerous cells have an abnormal cell cycle; something disrupts the cycle. Cancer happens when cells somehow get the signal to grow and replicate when they should not. They do not get the signal to die.

---

1. E. Bianconi et al., "An Estimation of the Number of Cells in the Human Body," *Annals of Human Biology* 40, no. 6 (2013): 463–71.

To understand how and why cancer occurs, we must understand the roles that oncogenes, tumor suppressor genes, and free radicals play. *Oncogenes* are involved in normal cell growth and replication. However, they can also be turned on (activated) or changed (mutated) in ways that give a cell the signal to grow uncontrollably or cause a cell not to listen to the message to die. We all have oncogenes. But this does not mean that we all will develop cancer. There needs to be something in the environment—a trigger—that will activate or mutate our oncogenes.[2]

A loaded gun just sitting on a table is not automatically harmful. But that same gun becomes dangerous when someone picks it up and pulls the trigger. Think of the loaded gun as the oncogene, and think of the triggerman as the environmental process that causes the activation and mutation of the oncogene.

Tumor suppressor genes protect against cancer. They slow down cell growth, repair damage to

2. "Cancer Basics," American Cancer Society, Accessed November 4, 2015, http://www.cancer.org/cancer/cancerbasics/index.htm.

cells, and tell cells when they need to die. When tumor suppressor genes become inactivated or fail to work properly, this can lead to the development of cancer as well.

Free radicals are molecules or parts of a cell that are unstable. Cells do not like to be unstable, so to become stable, free radicals interact with molecules of other cells that are stable. However, although this interaction stabilizes the former free radicals, the molecules they interacted with are now unstable and change into free radicals themselves. A chain reaction starts: Stable molecules become unstable, and normal molecules become free radicals. This can cause the disruption of a cell's normal cycle, leading a previously healthy cell to become cancerous

There are many different types of cancer. The affected body part or kind of tissue generally determines the name given. Cancer usually takes years to develop and be detected. It is important to understand that by the time cancer is detectable in the body, the process has been going on for several years, even decades. Many different things cause cancer, and I argue that the cause is usually multifactorial; that is, many factors are working together.

There is still much to learn about what causes cancer; research is ongoing. However, based on what we know, we can divide the causes of cancer into two broad groups: genetic, or inherited, and environmental, or lifestyle driven. Genetic mutations cause only a small percentage of cancers. Acquired genetic mutations account for the majority of cancer diagnoses.[3] It is usually exposure to something in the environment or a lifestyle choice that activates an oncogene, inactivates a tumor suppressor gene, or causes the production of free radicals.

Lifestyle habits such as tobacco smoking (resulting in exposure to firsthand and secondhand smoke),[4] excessive alcohol use, nutrient-deficient diets, low physical activity,[5] and excessive sun and

3. "Genetics and Cancer," American Cancer Society, Accessed November 6, 2015, http://www.cancer.org/cancer/cancercauses/geneticsandcancer/index.htm.
4. "Tobacco and Cancer," American Cancer Society, Accessed November 7, 2015, http://www.cancer.org/cancer/cancercauses/tobaccocancer/index.htm.
5. "Diet and Physical Activity," American Cancer Society, Accessed November 10, 2015, http://www.cancer.org/cancer/cancercauses/dietandphysicalactivity/index.htm.

UV radiation exposure[6] are all linked to cancer development. Some viruses, including HPV (human papilloma virus), hepatitis B, hepatitis C, Epstein-Barr virus (EBV), and HIV, are linked to certain types of cancer.[7]

A number of medical diagnostic tools and medications are also known to cause cancer, including X-rays, CT scans, drugs that suppress the immune system, various hormonal drugs, and certain cancer-treatment drugs. I know it sounds counterintuitive, but some chemotherapeutic drugs, as well as radiation therapy, are associated with the development of *second cancers*. These are cancers that may develop after treatment for a first, unrelated cancer. They are not the same as *recurrent cancers*, which return after treatment.[8]

---

6. "Sun and UV Exposure," American Cancer Society, Accessed November 10, 2015, http://www.cancer.org/cancer/cancercauses/sunanduvexposure/index.htm.

7. "Infectious Agents," American Cancer Society, Accessed November 10, 2015, http://www.cancer.org/cancer/cancercauses/othercarcinogens/infectiousagents/index.htm.

8. "Radiation Exposure and Cancer," American Cancer Society, Accessed November 11, 2015, http://www.cancer.org/cancer/cancercauses/radiationexposureandcancer/index.htm.

Many people are concerned that devices we commonly use may be carcinogenic—things like smart meters that measure the use of natural gas, water, and electricity in our homes. We're concerned about cosmetics, including skin moisturizers, perfumes, makeup, toothpaste, deodorants and antiperspirants, nail polish, shampoos and conditioners, and talcum powder. There's also concern about cell phones, cell-phone towers, fluoride, microwave ovens, household cleaners, and artificial sweeteners.[9] To date, there have been no definitive scientific studies proving that any of these cause cancer in humans.

A *carcinogen* is a substance or exposure that can lead to the development of cancer. However, not all carcinogens cause cancer in every person. In some instances, whether a carcinogen leads to cancer may depend on other factors, such as the length of time and intensity of the exposure or the person's genetic background. It's hard to know definitively if a carcinogen will cause cancer because it is unethical to carry out research that

---

9. "Other Carcinogens," American Cancer Society, Accessed November 12, 2015, http://www.cancer.org/cancer/cancercauses/othercarcinogens/index.htm.

intentionally exposes someone to a carcinogen and then wait to see if cancer develops. Usually, researchers find out that a carcinogen causes cancer in humans through a person's accidental, incidental exposure.

Most scientific research studies concerning carcinogens are done on lab animals or cell cultures, and it is not always clear whether the results will hold true for people. Due to the ethical and moral limitations mentioned previously, studies that involve people focus on questions about exposure to possible carcinogens rather than measuring cause and effect. Such studies are limited because people are exposed to many different things, at different times, and in many different environments (home, school, workplace, etc.) Additionally, it usually takes many years from exposure to a carcinogen to the time cancer is diagnosed, and people may not recall all the information about their exposure.[10] All of these factors make it very hard to say that any one particular exposure or sub-

---

10. "General Information about Carcinogens," American Cancer Society, Accessed November 14, 2015, http://www.cancer.org/cancer/cancer-causes/othercarcinogens/generalinformationaboutcarcinogens/index.htm.

stance caused cancer. Consequently, many studies are inconclusive.

So here is the main question: Just because the current research does not prove that a suspected carcinogen leads to cancer, does this necessarily mean that a relationship does not exist? Should we take the risk? Isn't it better, within reason, to err on the side of caution? I think it is. What do you think?

Causes of Cancer

A. Inherited cancers: genetic mutation (5–10 percent of cases)
  - Certain types of breast and ovarian cancer
  - Certain types of colon cancer
B. Acquired cancers (majority of cases)
  - Environmental exposures
  - Smoking
  - Infection (HPV, hepatitis B, hepatitis C, EBV, HIV)
  - Excessive alcohol use

- Medical tests (radiation from X-rays, CT scans)
- Lack of physical activity
- Medical treatments (chemotherapy, radiation)
- Poor diet
- Excessive exposure to sun and UV radiation

CHAPTER 2

THE "BIG C": IS CANCER REALLY THAT BIG OF A DEAL?

BECAUSE CANCER IS the second leading cause of death in the United States, it is a big deal. However, let's talk about how this disease affects people of Afro-Caribbean descent in particular. In the United States, the black population is not evenly spread out. According to the US Census Bureau, most of the black people living in the United States reside in New York and in Southern states, including Florida, Georgia, North Carolina, Virginia, and Maryland. Fifty-three percent of the black persons living in the United States but born in another country are from the Caribbean.[11] This number may be an understatement because the information is usually collected on a volunteer basis, and some individuals may choose not to participate for fear that

---

11 "2010 Census Summary File," United States Census Bureau, last modified December 21, 2015, http://census.gov/2010census.

the information collected may somehow be used to support deportation back to the Caribbean.

Studies have shown that members of minority groups in America have overall health statistics that are worse than those of whites. Significant health disparities exist when it comes to cancer and the black community. Blacks are more likely to be diagnosed with cancer in the very advanced stage of the disease, when options for treatment are limited and less likely to work. Compared to whites, blacks also have lower cancer survival rates. Studies show that black males are diagnosed with cancer more and are more likely to die of cancer than their white counterparts. Black females are diagnosed less often, but once diagnosed, are more likely to die than their white counterparts.[12]

The reasons for such health disparities continue to be a significant topic of research, but they are likely due to many different factors

12. "Cancer Facts & Figures for African Americans 2013–2014," American Cancer Society, last modified 2013, http://www.cancer.org/acs/groups/content/@epidemiologysurveilance/documents/document/acspc-036921.pdf.

interacting at the same time. These factors include a nutrient-poor diet; obesity; chronic stress; exposure to known carcinogens; excess exposure to tobacco and alcohol; lack of physical activity; and lack of adequate health insurance for essential preventive, early screening, and treatment services.

Because it is a silent killer, chronic stress deserves a bit more attention. Chronic stress leads to the constant production of stress hormones. Stress in and of itself is not a bad thing until it becomes a constant issue. In response to an urgent or immediate need, stress hormones, such as cortisol, epinephrine, and norepinephrine can be very beneficial to the body's overall health. With chronic stress, however, these same hormones are produced constantly, and this can play a role in the development of many health issues, including cancer. Chronic stress raises blood sugar levels (leading to diabetes), raises blood pressure (leading to hypertension and heart disease), and weakens the immune system (promoting the development of cancer). Unfortunately, many people are faced with constant stress due to home-life and workplace issues. People of color face additional stress due to discrimination because of the color of our skin. Despite advancements in many areas, people of color and other minorities are still forced to deal with this issue. Chronic stressors include perceived discrimination and racism, poverty, and family dysfunction.[13]

Some may view these factors as things that an individual can personally control, and that may be true in some cases. However, in many instances, such factors may be systematically perpetuated and therefore beyond any individual's control. Some factors are community based and environmental, including negative marketing strategies that target certain populations; lack of access to quality, nutrient-rich food; and fewer opportunities for physical activity. For example, in my community, there is a surplus of fast-food chain restaurants, limited access to truly organic foods, and an abundance of liquor stores. Alarmingly high numbers of people are uninsured and underinsured. Studies have also shown that people who believe they have experienced forms of discrimination or

---

13. "Fact Sheet: Health Disparities and Stress," American Psychological Association, last modified 2011, http://www.apa.org/topics/health-disparities/fact-sheet-stress.aspx/.

racism may be more likely to engage in unhealthy lifestyle behaviors such as poor nutrition choices; inadequate physical activity; abuse of tobacco, alcohol, and illicit substances; and improper use of available health-care services.

Religious beliefs may also play a role in cancer statistics. Some of my clients believe that their cancer diagnoses are forms of punishment God has implemented because of their wrongdoing. Others see their cancer as God's way of testing how strong their faith is, similar to what the prophet Job experienced. In either case, they are convinced that the cure is divine only—not to be found in traditional medicine at all. Such clients seek little or no medical care, and their adherence to recommendations by oncologists or other physicians may be minimal. Their solution is to pray and repent for their sins. This spiritual process may also include rituals such as prolonged, excessive fasting, which may further damage their health. Periodic or intermittent fasting may be beneficial to one's health by decreasing inflammation, decreasing cholesterol levels, lowering blood pressure, improving the health of the heart, decreasing the risk for diabetes by improving insulin sensitivity, improving immune system function, and triggering stem cell regeneration. Prolonged excessive fasting, however, done without a physician's supervision may result in adverse health effects, including dehydration, headache, dizziness, disrupted sleep patterns, memory problems, mental confusion, heartburn, fatigue, *hypotension* (dangerously low blood pressure), and *arrhythmias* (abnormal heart rhythms). Prolonged fasting may also put increased stress on the body, leading to the production of increased stress hormones. Other adverse effects include a weakened immune system as well as liver, kidney, and heart damage. With the combination of these factors in play, it is not surprising the effect that cancer is having on my community and other similar ones.[14]

In addition to the many underlying risk factors mentioned above, I can't help but wonder how the toxins in the dust after the terrorist attack on September 11, 2001, affected the cancer rates in my community. The dust contained many carcinogenic agents. It is a known fact that many first

---

14 Honor Whiteman, "Fasting: Health Benefits and Risks," Medical News Today (MNT), last updated July 27, 2015, www.medicalnewstoday.com/articles/295914.php/.

responders, as well as people who lived or worked nearby, were later diagnosed with cancer. My community is located near the site of the World Trade Center; it's just a ten-to-fifteen-minute walk from the World Trade Center to the Brooklyn Bridge, which connects Manhattan to the borough of Brooklyn. We know that cancer may take decades to develop, so although the attack took place more than ten years ago, we have yet to understand the full scope of the impact it may have on cancer rates, especially for neighboring communities like mine.

Both private and government-funded agencies have put in place many ongoing efforts to address and reduce the burden of cancer that disproportionately affects people of color. However, I do not believe that these efforts address the significant cultural differences that exist within the black population as a whole. Our cultural backgrounds are not homogenous. There is a major drawback to looking at health statistics based mainly on racial groupings without taking ethnicity and cultural norms more into account.

CHAPTER 3

"Let Food Be Your Medicine": Cancer and Our Food

Hippocrates, the Greek physician who is considered the father of modern medicine, is famous for saying, "Let food be thy medicine, and let medicine be thy food." Food is meant to do more than fill our bellies. The right combinations of nutrient-rich foods can be healing to our bodies and can help prevent and treat cancer. However, it is often difficult to know which foods to choose. Despite what you may have heard, no one food or nutrient will prevent or heal cancer. Nutrients do not exist in a bubble; they work together in a *synergistic* fashion. This means that the combined benefit is larger than the sum of the individual benefits. The interaction of many different nutrients in the right balance is most important.

Free radicals can be harmful to our cells in many ways, and they have been shown to play a role in the development of many disorders, including cancer. Yet free radicals are produced in many of the typical healthy reactions that take place in our bodies. Not only are they impossible to avoid; they are also necessary for optimal health. Free radicals help us fight off infection and start acute inflammatory reactions that our bodies need in order to repair injuries to our cells and tissues.[15]

On the flip side, having too many free radicals is not a good thing. I described the adverse health effects of chronic stress in the previous chapter. Chronic stress leads to increased free-radical production in the body. Exposure to environmental toxins such as those found in tobacco smoke, for example, also causes the body to produce more free radicals. The same holds true for excessive alcohol consumption. Moderate alcohol consumption may provide some health benefits. According to the Dietary Guidelines for Americans and the National Institute on Alcohol Abuse and Alcoholism, moderate alcohol consumption for men is defined as drinking up to

15. V. Lobo et al., "Free Radicals, Antioxidants, and Functional Foods: Impact on Human Health," *Pharmacognosy Reviews* 4, no. 8 (2010): 118–26.

two standard drinks per day. For women, moderate alcohol consumption is defined as drinking up to one standard drink per day. A standard drink contains about fourteen grams of alcohol. However, it is important to keep in mind that there are certain circumstances where drinking less may be considered excessive. For instance, if you have liver or heart disease, or are taking medications that negatively interact with alcohol, even one drink may be considered excessive.[16] Several reasons explain why the alcohol limits are set lower for women than for men. In general, women usually weigh less and have less water in their bodies than men have, which means there is less water in which alcohol is dispersed and less tissue to absorb the alcohol. Women usually have less of the enzyme (alcohol dehydrogenase) that breaks down alcohol. This allows the alcohol to remain in the system longer. Hormonal factors may also play a role, since some research studies suggest that blood alcohol levels are highest just

---

16 "Drinking Levels Defined," National Institute on Alcohol Abuse and Alcoholism, last modified April 2016, http://www. niaaa.nih.gov/alcohol-health/overview-alcohol-consumption/ moderate-binge-drinking.

prior to menstruation and lowest on the first day of menstruation.[17]

In addition to various pollutants present in the air we breathe, the water we drink, and the food we eat, ultraviolet (UV) radiation from the sun causes free radical formation. Prolonged sun exposure causes DNA mutations and is responsible for the majority of skin cancers. While it is true that people with lighter skin, due to less melanin, have a higher risk for skin cancer, it is still important to keep in mind that those with darker skin are at risk for cancer as well. Melanin is the pigment that is responsible for skin color and helps protect the skin from sun damage and skin cancer. There is a misconception that persons with more melanin are immune to skin cancer. It is this misconception that may be responsible for the fact that people with darker skin are diagnosed with skin cancer in later stages. Some reports suggest that this is what happened to the iconic reggae artist, Bob Marley. He died at thirty-six years of age, from a rare, aggressive form

---

17 "Why Is the Alcohol Limit Lower for Women?" Christian Nordqvist, Medical News Today, last modified December 4, 2015, http://www.medicalnewstoday.com/articles/265799.php#why_is_the_alcohol_limit_lower_for_women.

of melanoma skin cancer that started in his toe, but was initially dismissed as a soccer injury.[18]

Although prolonged exposure to the sun has been proven to be harmful, some studies suggest that moderate exposure (no more than 15–20 minutes per day) can have beneficial health effects, including bone health. Sunlight is required for the body to make vitamin D. Sunlight enhances mood and energy levels, kills bad bacteria, and increases the production of nitric oxide (NO), which in turn promotes the health of the cardiovascular system, promotes wound healing, and helps protect the skin against UV damage. UV radiation is also used to treat neonatal jaundice and various skin conditions including, eczema, acne, psoriasis, and vitiligo.[19]

The foods we eat may also be contributing to our overall cancer risk. Compared to whole foods, processed foods cause more free radicals

---

18 Mona Gohara and Marita Perez, "Skin Cancer and Skin of Color," Skin Cancer Foundation, last modified May 6, 2009, http://www.skincancer.org/prevention/skin-cancer-and-skin-of-color.

19 A. Juzeniene and M. Johan, "Beneficial Effects of UV Radiation Other Than via Vitamin D Production," *Dermato-Endocrinology* 4, no. 2 (2012): 109–17.

to develop in our bodies. Saturated and trans fats also produce free radicals more readily than the healthier unsaturated fats. Reading the nutrition labels on our food is crucial. If the term "partially hydrogenated oil" is listed in the ingredient list, we should do our best not to eat it because this is a trans fat.

Pesticides and herbicides are commonly used to protect our crops from insects, weeds, and diseases caused by fungi. Some farmers believe that without these chemicals, crop production would be significantly reduced because weeds often compete with crops for such natural resources as space, sunlight, water, and nutrients. Insects and diseases can eat away, destroy, or make our crops harder to grow and preserve long enough to reach our dining-room tables. However, the herbicides and pesticides commonly found in the food we eat can cause more free-radical formation.

According to research done by the Environmental Working Group (EWG), nearly two-thirds of the more than three thousand produce samples tested by the US Department of Agriculture in 2013 contained pesticides. The pesticides remained on the produce despite being washed and, in particular cases, despite being peeled. To help consumers make informed choices, the EWG has developed two helpful lists: the Dirty Dozen and the Clean Fifteen. The Dirty Dozen is a list of produce that contains the highest pesticide residues. Apples are number one; peaches, nectarines, strawberries, sweet bell peppers, cucumbers, cherry tomatoes, imported snap peas, and potatoes make the list as well. The Clean Fifteen are those fruits and vegetables with the least pesticides. Avocados are the cleanest; also included on the list are pineapples, onions, asparagus, mangoes, eggplant, cantaloupe, cauliflower, and kiwis.[20]

Dirty Dozen (ranked from most to least pesticide residue, dirtier to cleaner produce)

1. Apples
2. Peaches
3. Nectarines
4. Strawberries

---

20. "EWG's 2015 Shopper's Guide to Pesticides in Produce," Environmental Working Group, last modified February 25, 2015, http://www.ewg.org/foodnews/summary.php.

5. Grapes
6. Celery
7. Spinach
8. Sweet bell peppers
9. Cucumbers
10. Cherry tomatoes
11. Snap peas (imported)
12. Potatoes

Clean Fifteen (ranked from least to most pesticide residue, cleaner to dirtier produce)

1. Avocados
2. Sweet corn
3. Pineapples
4. Cabbage
5. Sweet peas (frozen)
6. Onions
7. Asparagus
8. Mangos
9. Papayas
10. Kiwi
11. Eggplant
12. Grapefruit
13. Cantaloupe

14. Cauliflower
15. Sweet potatoes

Although scientific studies about the human health risks of genetically engineered foods and food containing GMOs (genetically modified organisms) are inconclusive at this point, there is great concern about negative health effects.

Foods containing GMOs are not naturally occurring. They are created in a laboratory process known as *gene splicing*, where a gene from one species is put into another. This process makes the food longer lasting and more resistant to the effects of herbicides and pesticides. The most common GMO foods are corn and soy. Our meats are also of concern because cows, chickens, pigs, and farm-raised fish are often fed a diet made from GMOs.

In my opinion, it is best to err on the side of caution and consume as few GMO foods as possible. If possible, purchase foods labeled "non-GMO" or "GMO-free." It is often very difficult to avoid eating GMO foods because the law does not require that foods be labeled "GMO" or "GE."[21] It is best to read food labels carefully; eat meats from grass-fed animals; and buy organic, locally grown foods from farmers' markets.

For members of my community, this is tough to do because we have limited access to foods from the above sources. We often have to go elsewhere to find them, and even when they are available nearby, they are often much more expensive than other foods. I have also noticed that the healthier foods available in my community are priced higher than in those areas not populated by persons of color.

Even when the ideal situation exists—if we have consistent access to high-quality, nutrient-rich, organic foods that are grown without chemicals—these foods may contain herbicides, pesticides, and fungicides due to contamination of the soil, water, and air. So although potentially better than conventionally grown food, organic food may not really be organic. To be classified as a certified organic farmer, a grower simply has to provide a

---

21. "Non-GMO Shopping Guide," Institute for Responsible Technology, updated quarterly, http://www.nongmoshoppingguide.com.

written plan and documents to an inspector who does annual audits. These inspections, which are usually not surprises (unlike those in the restaurant business), generally involve reviewing documents and conducting baseline checks of the farms—but not gathering soil and crop samples to test for residues. So, in essence, this system is void of checks and balances and depends heavily on farmers being ethical, moral, and truthful.

A report in March 2010 by the US Department of Agriculture (USDA) Inspector General's office confirmed instances in which food labeled as "organic" did not comply with the standards—and instances in which companies were selling conventionally grown foods under the organic label. The report also showed that oversight was an issue. The USDA did not act fast enough to address loopholes and enforce regulations to ensure compliance with the standards for operation of organic farms.[22]

But how can you tell if your food is organic if it is not labeled? If we are referring to produce, a

---

22. "Oversight of the National Organic Program," USDA Office of the Inspector General, Audit Report 01601-03-HY, last modified March 2010, https://www.usda.gov/oig/webdocs/01601-03-HY.pdf.

useful way is to look at the PLU code. Have you ever wondered what that number sticker on that apple or orange means? It is called the *PLU code*. The PLU (Price Look-Up) code is a set of four- or five-digit numbers placed on produce. The cashier enters this code into the cash register at checkout to obtain the price. The code, assigned by the International Federation of Produce Standards (IFPS), is designed to make the checkout process and inventory control easy, fast, and accurate. However, use of the PLU code is voluntary, so some merchants might not use it. If the code has four digits and begins with a three or four, this means that the produce was conventionally grown (with the use of chemicals, herbicides, pesticides, and fungicides). If the code has five digits and starts with a nine, this means that the produce was organically grown.[23]

Because free radicals, if produced in excess, can cause DNA mutations that lead cells to become cancerous, we need to put a process in place that will neutralize free radicals. Antioxidants come

---

23. "Produce IFPS PLU Codes: A User's Guide," International Federation for Produce Standards, last modified Spring 2015, http://www.ifpsglobal.com/identification/PLU-codes.com/htm/.

into play here. *Antioxidants* are nutrients in whole foods that decrease or prevent the adverse health effects that free radicals have in our bodies. They can actually help repair and reverse the damage done. Adding antioxidants to our daily diet gives us an extra insurance policy for cancer prevention and healing. There are many different antioxidants, and the available research is still nowhere near complete enough to identify them all and define the full scope of all their health benefits.

However, some antioxidants are well known, including selenium; zinc; and vitamins A, C, and E. *Phytochemicals* are another classification of antioxidants. You can find phytochemicals in many different fruits, vegetables, and grains. Examples include flavonoids, polyphenols, lycopene, lutein, lignin, coenzyme Q (ubiquinone), glutathione, and superoxide dismutase.[24]

Because it can be very confusing to figure out if you are consuming antioxidant-rich foods, it is best to make sure you include lots of whole fruits

---

24. "Antioxidants 101," Gloria Tsang, HealthCastle.com, last modified March 1, 2011, http://www.healthcastle.com/antioxidant.shtml/.

and vegetables with bright and dark colors in great variety. Nuts are also rich in antioxidants. Tea, especially green tea, contains catechin, another kind of antioxidant.

CHAPTER 4

CONVENTIONAL APPROACHES TO CANCER PREVENTION AND TREATMENT

TRADITIONAL OR CONVENTIONAL methods for cancer prevention involve actions such as following the recommended screening exams and tests provided by your primary-care physician and adopting a healthy lifestyle. These healthy lifestyle practices include healthy eating, regular exercise, stress management, and avoidance of proven carcinogenic agents.

Cancer can be treated in many different ways and traditionally involves a team of doctors and medical professionals who specialize in cancer treatment. The type of treatment chosen usually depends on the particular type of cancer. For example, breast-cancer treatment is different from lung- or stomach-cancer treatment. The treatment plan will also depend on other factors, including the stage of the disease, the progression of the cancer, and the overall health of the individual diagnosed. In some cases, a combination of traditional treatments is used.

The goals of cancer-treatment regimens also vary from cure to comfort. Most treatments are designed with a cure in mind. However, in some cases, when cure is not possible due to the type, stage, or location of cancer, treatment plans may relieve pain and other symptoms of cancer, thereby possibly improving the quality of life remaining. There are numerous cancer-treatment options, and research is ongoing. However, the most common types of traditional cancer treatments are chemotherapy, radiation, surgery, stem-cell transplant, hormonal therapy, and immunotherapy. A brief overview of each of these common types is outlined below.

Chemotherapy, or chemo, refers to medications used to kills cancer cells, prevent cancer from spreading, and relieve the symptoms of cancer. It is usually given intravenously, through a catheter placed in the vein. It may also be given into the muscle or by mouth. Because most chemotherapeutic drugs are very strong, they are usually given in cycles—short periods of treatments followed by a recovery period to give the body a rest. Chemotherapy is commonly used when doctors believe that cancer has already spread from the place where it originally started. It works by killing the cancer cells that have spread, or *metastasized*, to other parts of the body. Chemotherapy may be used alone or with other forms of treatment. For example, given before surgery, chemotherapy can shrink tumors and make them easier to remove. Chemo may also be given after surgery to kill any cancer cells that may have been left behind.[25]

Surgery can be used to prevent, diagnose, stage, and treat cancer. When prevention is the goal, tissue may be removed because it is precancerous and likely to become cancerous. A good example of this is when polyps are removed from the colon during a colonoscopy. Surgery used for diagnosis generally refers to a *biopsy*, a procedure in which a piece of tissue believed to be cancerous is removed and tested to see if it contains cancerous cells. When used to determine

---

25. "Chemotherapy Basics," American Cancer Society, http://www.cancer.org/treatment/treatmentsandsideeffects/treatmenttypes/chemotherapy/index.

the stage of cancer that a patient has, surgery seeks to determine whether and how much a cancer has spread. Surgery may be used as the only form of treatment when the cancer is confined to a particular location. During the surgical procedure, the cancerous areas, as well as surrounding tissues and lymph nodes, are removed. In some advanced cases, however, cancer cannot be removed without damage to neighboring healthy tissues or organs. So surgery may be used before other treatments to eliminate some cancerous cells.[26]

Radiation involves using high-energy waves to kill cancer cells. Radiation damages the DNA of cancerous cells so that they are no longer able to grow and rapidly divide. This causes the cancerous cells to die. Radiation may be used alone or in combination with other traditional treatments. For example, after surgery, radiation may get rid of any cancerous cells left behind after the surgical procedure. Like surgery, radiation is

26. "A Guide to Cancer Surgery," American Cancer Society, http://www.cancer.org/treatment/treatmentsandsideeffects/treatmenttypes/surgery/index.

used mainly for cancers confined to one region of the body.[27]

Stem-cell transplant is another form of cancer treatment used to replace and restore stem cells destroyed or damaged by underlying cancer or by other treatments. *Stem cells* are the immature cells that live mainly in the bone marrow. These cells eventually mature, leave the bone marrow for the bloodstream, and become red blood cells, white blood cells, or platelets. Red blood cells carry oxygen to all the cells in the body; white blood cells fight infection. Platelets help stop bleeding by forming healthy blood clots. Stem-cell transplants are often used after other cancer treatments and are often given intravenously. The goal is for the transplanted cells to grow and mature in the bone marrow and leave the bone marrow for the bloodstream as healthy new cells. The cells used for the transplant can come from an identical twin, a close family member, or even, in some cases, the person with the cancer diagnosis. Before the

27. "Radiation Therapy," American Cancer Society, http://www.cancer.org/treatment/treatmentsandsideeffects/treatmenttypes/radiation/index.

individual starts cancer treatment, the stem cells are removed and preserved for later use.[28]

Hormonal therapy is useful in certain cancers that are hormonally dependent. This mode of treatment involves the use of medications that lower the production of certain hormones or the removal of the particular organs that produce them. Hormonal therapy works best for certain cancers of the breast, testicle, and prostate.[29]

Immunotherapy, also called "biological therapy," is very effective for certain types of cancer and, in general, is designed to make the immune system stronger and more effective at killing cancer cells. It involves the use of medications that cause the body's natural immune system to work better—or the use of synthetic versions of proteins naturally found in the immune system. Immunotherapy

---

28. "Stem Cell Transplant (Peripheral Blood, Bone Marrow, and Cord Blood Transplants)," American Cancer Society, http://www.cancer.org/treatment/treatmentsandsideeffects/treatmenttypes/bonemarrowandperipheralbloodstemcelltransplant/index.

29. "Hormone Therapy," American Cancer Society, http://www.cancer.org/cancer/cancer-treating-hormone-therapy/index.

may be used alone or in combination with other cancer treatments.[30]

Many people are very concerned about the side effects of different cancer treatments, and rightfully so. In medicine, the term *side effects* is usually used to describe a negative or unintended consequence that a drug, medical procedure, or medical treatment can have on the individual. There are many different side effects of cancer treatments, some physical and others emotional. The side effects may vary from person to person, depending on the type of cancer treatment used, the intensity of the treatment, how frequently it is given, and the route used to give it (intravenous or oral). Most cancer treatments destroy normal cells as well as cancerous cells. The destruction often leads to an increase of toxins and cell waste, which can result in side effects.

Nausea, vomiting, and fatigue are some of the most common side effects of chemo and radiation therapy. Other known side effects of

---

30. "Cancer Immunotherapy," American Cancer Society, http://www.cancer.org/treatment/treatmentsandsideeffects/treatmenttypes/immunotherapy/index.

cancer treatments include *anemia* (low red-blood-cell count), *neutropenia* (low white-blood-cell count), and *thrombocytopenia* (low platelet count). Neutropenia increases the chance of developing an infection because the white blood cells are important elements of the immune system. *Lymphedema* is another common side effect that can occur after surgery or radiation therapy. Lymphedema is the buildup of lymphatic drainage under the skin that occurs because of damage to the lymphatic system. The lymphatic system is important because it contains nodes that filter toxic substances from the body. Pain is another common side effect of various cancer treatments. For instance, chemotherapy and radiation may cause damage to the nerves, leading to peripheral neuropathy. Symptoms include pain, tingling, burning, numbness, and weakness in the hands and feet. Cancer treatments also can result in sexual dysfunction and infertility in both men and women.[31]

The side-effect profile scares many people and leads them to avoid conventional methods for dealing with cancer. The quality of life is of utmost

31. "Treatments and Side Effects," American Cancer Society, http://www.cancer.org/treatment/treatmentsandsideeffects/index.htm.

importance. People are not willing to accept the idea of not being able to carry on with their daily activities and not being able to enjoy life in general. Many people suffer needlessly because they are resistant to using traditional approaches due to the side effects. As a physician, I understand the role that conventional methods of cancer treatment play in healing, but I also know that more needs to be done so that patients with cancer can become truly cancer free. The conventional methods are excellent in the acute setting. However, they are not best for prevention and real healing. It is important to understand that conventional cancer treatments have their place and are of great use once cancer is diagnosed.

However, while the conventional approaches to cancer prevention and treatment may work well for some in other communities, they have often been great disappointments for members of my community and similar communities. Approaches like these do not adequately address the problem; a more comprehensive, holistic approach is required. A big piece of the puzzle is missing. The goals of this book are to discuss why conventional approaches do not always work and present what I believe that missing piece to be.

But before revealing the missing piece, let's recap why the currently used guidelines and practices for cancer prevention and treatment are not enough, particularly for those in my community:

- Unhealthy lifestyle habits
- Lack of regular access to fresh, unprocessed, whole foods
- Presence of high amounts of herbicides and pesticides in our foods
- Lack of access to truly organic foods
- Living in the post-9/11 era, very close to ground zero
- Being uninsured or underinsured, which prevents early detection through screening
- Chronic stress
- Unique cultural beliefs and norms
- Religious beliefs that delay accessing health-care services
- Health disparities—inequalities concerning health-care issues that are seemingly based on race, ethnicity, income, immigration status, and so on

Now that we have looked at some of the causes of cancer in humans, let's look at a proven solution, which is the focus of the second part of this book.

PART 2

THE SOLUTION

CHAPTER 5

Eating Right May Not Be Enough: A More Holistic Approach to Cancer Prevention and Treatment

I WOULD LIKE to see my patients develop and use a system of wellness that can help conventional methods of cancer treatment work optimally. This wellness system should protect against the many side effects of various conventional cancer treatments and should be effective at keeping cancer survivors free of cancer. Ideally, however, this wellness system should be used as the ultimate prevention strategy. It should be used to prevent cancer before it even starts. Again, a prevention strategy should include stress management, avoiding tobacco and excessive alcohol consumption, healthy physical activity, and healthy eating.

In my opinion, one major problem for people who live in a community like mine is the lack of proper nutrition to nourish, cleanse, and protect the body. The solution is quality nutrition supplementation. When I use the term *nutrition supplementation*, I am referring to the use of vitamins, minerals, antioxidants, and other nutrients that have been put in powder, pill, or liquid form for daily use. Supplements should not replace healthy eating and other healthy lifestyle habits but should be used along with them.

When I was in medical school, I was taught that if we "ate right," there was no need for nutritional supplements. I learned that our food had all that we needed to keep the body healthy, so it was not necessary to look elsewhere to complete our nutritional needs. I used to believe that all these nutritional-supplement companies were just out to make a buck, enticing consumers to purchase all different forms of dietary supplements. I used to think that these supplements would not enhance anyone's health and, in some cases, could cause harm. However, based on my personal experience and my professional experience as a health coach, I now believe that nutritional supplements, used in the right manner, can be a very useful addition to an existing wellness program.

Like me, most physicians don't get adequate training in nutrition and how to use nutrients to prevent disease and heal the body. In medical school, we learn about the importance of a few basic nutrients. We know about the B vitamins as well as vitamins A, C, D, and K. We're familiar with folate, iron, calcium, magnesium, and the omegas. But beyond the very basics, most of us lack the knowledge to counsel our patients further on these and the many other nutrients that are essential for optimal health. Most physicians are taught mainly how to diagnose and treat a disease or illness once it has developed, using pharmaceuticals and surgical procedures.

Please do not misunderstand me: Medication and surgery are an important part of health care. But it is important to keep in mind that any conventional approach to health care will be more effective if a person has a great nutritional foundation. It was not until I went back to school to earn my degree in public health and my certification as a health coach that I started to understand the enormous role that nutrition plays in achieving and maintaining optimal health and wellness.

Some research suggests that the body needs as much as ninety nutrients daily to be at an optimal level of wellness and function. Due to processing techniques, biotechnology methods, contamination, food allergies, seasonal availability of certain foods, personal preferences, and poor dietary habits, we are no longer getting what we used to get from our food. In essence, there exists an enormous gap between what we get in the food we eat daily and what our bodies need to be healthy.

How do we bridge this gap? The answer is to supplement the diet using nutrients in the right proportion and balance. Supplementation is a quick, easy, and efficient way to get what is supposed to be in our food but is not. It is an excellent option for those who do not have regular access to high-quality, whole, unprocessed foods. Supplementation helps cleanse and protect the body from the negative properties in our foods and in our environments, which can play a role in the development of cancer and other diseases. In our community, located just minutes from the site of the World Trade Center attacks, supplementation is necessary to provide various nutrients that are known to fight and prevent cancer. If used in the right way, supplementation will not only lessen the side effects of conventional cancer treatments but will also help these treatments work better.

CHAPTER 6

NOT ALL SUPPLEMENTS ARE CREATED EQUAL: HOW TO CHOOSE

ONCE YOU UNDERSTAND how quality nutritional supplements play a role in the prevention and healing of cancer, the learning process does not stop. Now you have to choose which supplement(s) to use, and that can be a daunting and challenging task. There are many different lines of supplements available on the market. Some are good, some not so good.

It is important to bear in mind that nutritional supplements are not meant to replace any medication that physicians prescribe. If your doctor has prescribed medication for you, please take it. A great concern for many patients is that supplements may interact negatively with prescription medications. But quality nutritional supplements are designed to make prescription drugs work better and also to protect the body from the negative side effects of prescription medications. I want to make it clear that using supplements should not be a substitute for good medical care. I urge patients to work with a health care provider knowledgeable about nutrition in general, as well as nutritional supplements to ensure that the regimen being used for supplementation is beneficial and not interfering with any medications that have been prescribed. In my holistic health practice, I guide patients by helping them decide which supplements to add to their daily wellness plans. I have personally seen cases in which patients have been able to take lower dosages of their medications several months after starting to use the supplements I recommended.

I believe that the right nutritional supplements can also play a role in primary cancer prevention by protecting the body from the adverse effects of free radicals, preventing cell damage, assisting in cell repair, preventing the activation of oncogenes, and promoting necessary programmed cell death. For a person with a cancer diagnosis, the right nutritional supplements can support and augment the action of the various conventional cancer treatments and help protect the body from their harmful side effects. Quality supplements can also kick-start the body's innate mechanism for fighting cancer by strengthening the immune system. An active, well-functioning immune system is needed to fight cancer and kill cancerous cells.

What is the right nutritional supplement? Do the research!

Here is a list of factors to consider when choosing a nutritional supplement:

- **Choose balanced supplements.**
  - The right supplement is balanced and comprehensive, with the right proportion of nutrients: vitamins, minerals, trace elements, antioxidants, and digestive-enzyme support to enhance absorption. It should also contain the right dosages. Nutrients are designed to complement one another, and for one nutrient to exert its full effect on the body, several other nutrients are required.
  - During initial consultations with clients, I review what supplements, if any, they are using. Those who already use

supplements generally show me one to three bottles containing individual supplements—often calcium, vitamin D, and omega fatty acids or fish oil—and sometimes a multivitamin containing twenty-five to thirty vitamins, minerals, and essential nutrients. While this amount of nutrients may be enough to prevent major deficiencies, it is not sufficient to help achieve optimal health and wellness.

- **Choose supplements made in an FDA-approved lab using cGMP.**
  - One concern for many consumers is the lack of regulatory standards governing the practices by which some supplements are made. However, guidelines do exist. The term "cGMP" stands for "current good manufacturing practices." These are outlined by the US Food and Drug Administration (FDA) to ensure the appropriate monitoring, design, and control of the methods by which supplements are made and the facilities in which they are made. The cGMP regulations ensure that

supplements are of good quality by requiring manufacturers to use quality raw materials and ingredients. The cGMP also requires that top-notch systems and equipment are used to make supplements. In a nutshell, use of the cGMP makes sure that supplements are safe and free of contaminants, toxins, and impurities.[32]

- It is not a federal requirement that nutritional-supplement companies make their products in FDA-approved labs. The FDA is not authorized or required to review supplements for safety and efficacy before they are marketed. However, the FDA will take action against any supplement shown to be unsafe once it reaches the market. If the FDA can prove that a supplement company is making false claims about its products, the agency will take actions to remove those supplements from the market. I

32. "Facts about the Current Good Manufacturing Practices (CGMPs)," US Food and Drug Administration, last modified January 2015, http://www.fda.gov/Drugs/DevelopmentApprovalProcess/Manufacturing/ucm169105.htm.

recommend using supplements from a company that voluntarily makes its supplements in an FDA-approved lab because this provides another level of purity and quality control.[33]

- **Choose supplements with ingredients that are natural, in a whole food base, and free of herbicides and pesticides.**
- **Choose supplements with raw ingredients and nutrients that have GRAS designation.**
  - The FDA uses the GRAS ("generally recognized as safe") designation to let consumers know that a panel of experts considers the ingredients in a particular supplement to be safe for human consumption. GRAS designation can be self-affirmed— determined by the manufacturer using a predetermined set of specifications—or the FDA can be notified of GRAS determination by a nongovernmental outside expert.[34]

---

33. "FDA 101: Dietary Supplements," US Food and Drug Administration, http://www.fda.gov/ForConsumers/ConsumerUpdates/ucm050803. htm.

34. "Generally Recognized as Safe (GRAS)," US Food and Drug Administration, last modified June 2015, http://www.fda.gov/food/ ingredientspackaginglabeling/gras/.

- **Choose supplements from a reputable source or company.**
  - Select a company with a known track record that has been around for a substantial amount of time.
  - Choose a company that uses quality controls and standards that surpass even those required by the FDA.
- **Make sure you can easily use and introduce your chosen supplements into your daily routine.**
  - Supplements can be of high quality and efficacy, but they will work for you only if you use them on a regular basis. My clients often complain that they have difficulty remembering to take their supplements every day. Most of us lead busy lives, so we need to find a way to introduce our supplements seamlessly into our daily routines. This is why I suggest setting an alarm as a reminder. Using a liquid supplement is great for my patients who use prescription medications that are in a pill/capsule form and are not excited about the idea of adding more pills/capsules to their wellness

plan. Liquid supplements are also of benefit to people who find it hard to swallow pills or capsules.

- **Consider the formulation (liquid, powder, capsule, or tablet).**
  - It is also important to consider the formulation of supplements you choose. The main difference among these tends to be the absorption rate. Because liquids can be added to other liquids and powders can dissolved in liquids easily, they tend to be absorbed faster by the body. Another advantage of liquid or powder supplements is that they are easier to swallow than are capsules or tablets. However, some nutrients are not as stable in liquid form and must be put into tablet or capsule form to be active in the body. Capsules are usually easier to swallow than tablets.

- **Choose supplements that your body will absorb.**
  - Critics will tell you that nutritional supplements are ineffective because they are not absorbed by the body. In this view, the acidic environment of

the stomach destroys the nutrients in the supplements before they can be absorbed in the less acidic environment of the small intestine.

- If this is your concern, you may prefer to choose liquid supplements or enteric (coated) pills. Liquid supplements are generally better absorbed because they skip most processing in the digestive tract and go directly into the bloodstream. Enteric coating protects the supplement from stomach acids, allowing the nutrients in the tablet to get safely to the small intestine, where most of the absorption takes place. The coating also makes tablets easier to swallow and prevents the stomach upset that many people complain about after taking tablets. Enteric coating also allows for the slow or extended release of active ingredients, which in turn allows more time for absorption.

- **Pay attention to the "% DV" (percent of daily value).**
  - Many consumers are concerned about nutritional supplements that go above

the "% DV" listed on labels. There is concern about overdosing if a supplement exceeds the recommended DV.

- The "% DV" designation was developed to let consumers know how much of a particular nutrient is in that food or supplement. It helps us figure out if a food or supplement is high or low in nutrition. For example, if the label refers to 35 percent Daily Value for vitamin C, this means that one serving of that food or supplement contains 35 percent of the daily quantity of vitamin C that the FDA recommends.[35]

- It is important to keep in mind that the "% DV" refers to the *minimum* daily amount required to prevent a major deficiency in that nutrient. The "% DV" is usually not nearly enough for the body to reach optimal health and wellness. Additionally, if you have a particular medical problem and are taking a

---

35. "How to Understand and Use the Nutrition Facts Label," US Food and Drug Administration, last modified April 2015, http://www.fda.gov/Food/IngredientsPackagingLabeling/LabelingNutrition/ucm274593.htm.

prescription medication, your nutrient requirements are often much higher than those recommended by the FDA. If you are taking a beta blocker (high-blood-pressure medication), or statin (cholesterol-lowering medication), for example, this may increase your need for coenzyme Q, an antioxidant known to play a role in cardiovascular health. Another example is vitamin D. We all know the role vitamin D plays in bone health. However, there is abundant research suggesting other benefits. Being overweight has been linked to low vitamin D levels, suggesting that this group's requirements may be higher than those of normal-weight individuals. There are also some studies suggesting that vitamin D plays a role in preventing certain types of cancer. The DV for vitamin D is 600 IU (International Units) for people between the ages of four and seventy and 800 IU for those older than seventy-one. This quantity may be enough to prevent a major deficiency leading to rickets, osteomalacia (softening of the bones), or osteoporosis (weak or brittle bones), but studies suggest that much higher doses are required to take advantage of the other benefits of vitamin D (cancer prevention, cardiovascular health, a stronger immune system, improved cognition, and brain health).

CHAPTER 7

WHAT'S NEXT? WHERE DO YOU GO FROM HERE?

As a board-certified, licensed physician, I never thought I would write a book about the benefits of nutritional supplements. However, having worked with so many patients over more than a decade and having seen the benefits they received, it is too hard for me to keep the information to myself, especially when so many people are looking for help.

The primary goal of this book is to demonstrate the role that nutritional supplements can play in the prevention and healing of cancer. I believe supplements can be an essential part of an overall wellness program. The right supplement can augment the effects of prescription medications and can help protect the body from the harmful side effects of medications. However, because not all nutritional-supplement companies use comprehensive techniques to ensure the efficacy, quality, and safety of their supplements, it is difficult for the average consumer to be confident in deciding which supplements to use. If you choose to use nutritional supplements (and I hope after reading this book, you will), please do your research thoroughly and then consult with a trained professional who has the knowledge to help you in the decision-making process, especially when it comes to dealing with cancer.

As a physician and health coach with a master's degree in public health, I am in a unique position to help people develop easy-to-follow, safe, effective, and personalized wellness programs. These programs involve recommendations for healthy lifestyle modifications, with guidelines and techniques for stress management, such as meditation, positive spiritual affirmations, and referrals for psychological counseling when appropriate. The wellness programs that I help my patients design also include recommendations for the avoidance of known toxins and carcinogenic agents as well as healthy exercise and eating plans. The eating plans, of course, allow my patients to enjoy the well-known Caribbean favorites and staples. As outlined in part 1 of this book, because of various issues with the quality of our food, the wellness programs include suggestions for the use of nutritional supplements to bridge the existing nutritional gaps. I recommend supplements from one particular company that I have thoroughly researched. I am confident in the safety, quality, and effectiveness of these supplements. Following are few success stories.

Mary: Breast-Cancer Free in Six Months

Mary noticed a lump in her breast, and it was confirmed to be cancerous (stage II) by mammogram and tissue biopsy. She started using the supplements I recommended while waiting for a second opinion to reconfirm the diagnosis and start traditional cancer treatments. In six months, the lump in her breast had disappeared, and her oncologist informed her that she no longer had cancer and did not need any cancer treatment. She has continued using the supplements along with other healthy lifestyle habits as a preventive strategy. For the past seven years, Mary has continued to have normal breast exams and mammograms.

Joan: Improvement in Chemotherapy Side Effects

Joan was being treated with traditional chemotherapy for lymphoma, a type of blood-cell cancer involving the cells of the lymphatic system. The lymphatic system is part of the body's immune system and is comprised of cells that help the body to rid itself of toxins, waste, and other unwanted substances.[36] Joan's doctor discontinued chemotherapy because of her low white-blood-cell and red-blood-cell counts and her heart complications. The physician told her that these side effects were caused by her cancer medications. Because of their severity, nothing else could be done for her at that time. Her physician instructed her to start putting her affairs in order and prepare for the worst. As a last resort, Joan started the supplementation program I recommended. After three months, at a follow-up visit to her doctor, she was told that her counts were up, the health of her heart had improved, and she could start chemotherapy again.

---

36 "The Lymphatic System and Cancer," Cancer Research UK, last modified October 29, 2014, http://www.cancerresearchuk. org/about-cancer/what-is-cancer/body-systems-and-cancer/ the-lymphatic-system-and-cancer.

Robert: Cancer Stopped Spreading in Three Months

Robert was diagnosed with stage IV cancer, with significant spread to other organs, particularly the liver and kidney. Despite traditional chemotherapy, his cancer continued to spread. He started the supplements I recommended, and after three months, his doctors told him that his cancer had stopped spreading and that his liver and kidneys no longer showed evidence of cancer. He also had more energy and got the color back in his skin, which he noticed he had lost after starting chemotherapy.

Alicia: Improved Quality of Life Despite Cancer and Chemotherapy

Alicia was diagnosed with leukemia, a type of cancer involving the white blood cells. The white blood cells help the body fight off infections. Normally white blood cells grow, as needed, in an orderly fashion. However, in people with leukemia, the white blood cells are abnormally produced and do not function properly.[37] Alicia started chemo-

---

37 "Diseases and Conditions: Leukemia," Mayo Clinic, last modified January 28, 2016, http://www.mayoclinic.org/diseases-conditions/leukemia/basics/definition/con-20024914.

therapy for her leukemia and noticed that right after her treatment, she had little energy—she felt exhausted and weak. Alicia would be in bed the rest of the day after her chemo session and all of the next day, too, because it would take her that long to recover. After starting the supplements I recommended, she noticed that these symptoms subsided. She was able to get her cancer treatments and still be active in the days after her treatments. She even went bowling with her daughter, something she had not been able to do since her cancer diagnosis.

There are countless other success stories that I will never get the chance to collect and share, because these clients started using the supplements before a cancer diagnosis. In essence, they were able to prevent cancer—they were never diagnosed with cancer because they stopped it before it could develop.

CONCLUSION

A BURNING DESIRE to help my community prompt-
ed me to write this book. My community is com-
posed of people of Afro Caribbean descent and
other people of color living in post-9/11 urban areas with limited access to healthy food. I hope to
be an inspiration for others to participate actively
in healthy living. The first step is to acknowledge
the gaps that exist in our nutrition. The second
step is to understand and evaluate the reasons for
these gaps. The third and final step is to work with
a qualified health-care provider to find ways to
close these gaps. Cancer, being the second leading
cause of death in the United States, is much more
common today than in previous decades.[38] For
communities like mine, a nutrition supplementa-

38. "National Center for Health Statistics: Leading Causes of Death,"
Centers for Disease Control and Prevention (CDC), last modified
February 25, 2016, http://www.cdc.gov/nchs/fastats/leading-causes-
of-death.htm.

tion program plays a vital role by supporting traditional cancer-treatment programs, preventing cancer from developing, contributing to overall health and wellness, and improving the general quality of life.

In the end, it's not the years in your life that count. It's the life in your years.

—*Abraham Lincoln*

Each and every one of us has to find quality in our lives, and one of the main determinants of quality is health status. Cancer can have significant negative effects on quality of life. If my thoughts and views on preventing and healing cancer help one person, I feel my goal has been accomplished. Let's work together to end the cancer crisis. It starts with you!

If you are interested in learning more about the wellness programs I design, the nutritional supplements I recommend, or setting up a consultation, feel free to visit my website at www.drrhondacambridgephillip.com, fill out a "Contact Me" form, and leave a brief message. You may also call 917-601-7728.

Don't miss a single thing! Sign up for my newsletter for more interesting topics and information at www.drrhondacambridgephillip.com/newsletter.

Hire me to speak at your next event! I am very passionate about making a difference and eradicating nutritional suicide, one person at a time. I have been speaking to groups and organizations for more than ten years. I am an expert in the field and have spoken to hundreds of people in my community.

For more information, or to hire me for your next keynote presentation, please visit www.drrhondacambridgephillip.com, fill out a "Contact Me" form, and leave a brief message.

Did you enjoy this book? I would love your review. Please give me your honest feedback on my website or on Amazon.com.